Thorsons Complete Guide to Homoeopathically Prepared Mineral Tissue Salts

A clear and concis
most expert in the
therapy and how i
combat common a

G000076743

Thorsons Complete Guide to Homoeopathically Prepared Mineral Tissue Salts

Dr Peter Gilbert
B.A., M.B., B.S., M.R.C.S., L.R.C.P.

Thorsons
An Imprint of HarperCollinsPublishers

Thorsons
An Imprint of HarperCollins*Publishers*
77–85 Fulham Palace Road,
Hammersmith, London W6 8JB.

Published by Thorsons 1989
10 9 8 7 6 5 4 3

A catalogue record for this book
is available from the British Library

ISBN 0 7225 1942 7

Printed in Great Britain by
HarperCollinsManufacturing Glasgow

Contents

	Introduction	7
Chapter 1	A brief history of mineral tissue salts	9
Chapter 2	Mineral tissue salts in self-medication	11
Chapter 3	The single mineral tissue salts	16
Chapter 4	The combination mineral tissue salts	30
Chapter 5	How to use mineral tissue salts	35
Chapter 6	Care of the whole person	44
Chapter 7	Hints on the relief of hay fever	47
Chapter 8	Minerals and trace elements	54
Chapter 9	Therapeutic index	59
Chapter 10	Female conditions	67
Chapter 11	Therapeutic index for children	69
Chapter 12	Therapeutic index for pets	73
	Appendix	75
	Index	78

About the Author

Peter Gilbert, who qualified in medicine 40 years ago, is the leading expert on mineral tissue salt therapy. His father was the founder of the Schuessler Society and the British Biochemic Association, and Peter Gilbert learnt the art of using the mineral tissue salt treatment at an early age. He firmly believes that homoeopathically prepared mineral tissue salts offer a viable alternative to drugs for the treatment of everyday ailments.

He has a Harley Street practice, and is a Fellow of the Royal Society of Medicine, a Fellow and founder member of the Medical Acupuncture Society, a founder member of the Society of Hypnosis and a Liveryman of the Worshipful Society of Apothecaries.

Introduction

The last few years have seen a great change in the attitudes of the medical profession and the general public towards complementary medicine. There is now a considerable body of doctors who are prepared to acknowledge that complementary medicine works. Moreover, it works in a gentle way, does not have the side-effects increasingly associated with much drug therapy, and is non-addictive. If a patient benefits, then everyone should celebrate. Such a change in professional attitudes is very gratifying to me, since I have been championing the cause for over 40 years.

A number of common drugs, even aspirin, have recently been criticized for their side-effects and levels of safety. Naturally, this has concerned many people, and they have begun to look towards natural remedies for the treatment of illness.

There is, of course, a time and a place for both types of medicine. In my practice in Harley Street, I prescribe both when the occasion demands. However, in general I believe that it is wrong to prescribe an allopathic medicine when a natural remedy will be perfectly adequate. When you are considering self-help, then it is to the natural medicines that you should first turn.

Of all the methods of self-help available, the safest in my opinion is mineral tissue salt therapy. This book is about this therapy, what it is, how to use it and when to use it. I believe that no other system can compete with mineral tissue salts with their combination of simplicity and effectiveness.

I have written this book as a guide and reference for those who are thinking about mineral tissue salts for the first time, and those who wish to understand more about the subject. Homoeopathically prepared mineral tissue salts are more widely available than ever before. You will find them in health food stores and, increasingly, in pharmacies.

I have used mineral tissue salts extensively over the last 40 years, both in my medical practice and for myself. I can vouch for their efficacy in a great range of conditions. People, I feel, should help themselves; that is, with all due safeguard, take a hand in getting themselves well and keeping themselves well. That is the purpose of this book. I would like to acknowledge the invaluable help and assistance with research for this book from the New Era Company in the preparation of the information in it.

1 A brief history of mineral tissue salts

From the earliest days of medicine, mineral salts of various forms have been used. However, the system of mineral tissue salt medicine is credited to Dr Wilhelm Heinrich Schuessler, a man of great vision who was far ahead of his time.

Schuessler was born in 1821. After qualifying in medicine, he became interested in homoeopathy and received his licence to practise as a homoeopathic physician in the town of Oldenburg on the north German coast close to Hamburg. Homoeopathy was still in its infancy at that time. Samuel Hahnemann had completed his revolutionary work at Leipzig in the early years of that century. Schuessler was, therefore, an early adapter of this new system of medicine. At first he used the full range of homoeopathic medicines in his practice, but gradually he narrowed things down to the use of inorganic substances. Schuessler's imagination had been fired by the idea that the organs of the body depended upon necessary amounts of inorganic constituents for their structure and vitality. He predicted that these inorganic elements would prove to be central to the systems of medicine and agriculture. In the field of agriculture, his forecast has been fully fulfilled.

In March 1873 Dr Schuessler published *Shortened Therapeutics* in which he expounded his theories on body chemistry. This was later considerably expanded, by a series of articles, into the complete exposition of the mineral tissue salt therapy that we have today.

Schuessler's influence was extensive, both during his lifetime and after his death in 1898. A fellow German, Dr Julius Hensel, published various works on minerals in the 1880s, including a remarkable book *Bread from Stones*, which showed how grinding stones from a field into a fine powder and then returning the powder to the soil improved crop fertility. In England, the work on agricultural minerals was continued by my father, Dr Henry Gilbert, and at the Rothamsted Research Station.

The Schuessler salts were introduced to America by Dr H.C.G. Luyties of St Louis, Missouri, who had visited Schuessler in Oldenburg. He translated Schuessler's work into English. Later, Dr Constantine Hering of Philadelphia, one of the founders of homoeopathy in America, published a book on this system of medicine. A further important work on the *Schuessler Salts* was written by Dr M. Docetti Walker of Dundee, a woman I remember well from my childhood.

In 1911, the British Biochemic Association was founded under the patronage of the Earl of Dysort as the first President. My father, Dr Henry Gilbert, was made Vice-President for life. He had set up the Gilbert Laboratories in Grantham to manufacture the 12 Schuessler salts and some related products such as Biosalt. He also had a very busy medical practice, attracting clients from all over the world.

Dr Luyties also manufactured remedies in England at a plant in the town of Slough. This facility eventually grew into the New Era Company, which transferred to Park Royal in the London area before entering new custom-built facilities at Hull in October 1985.

The British Biochemic Association continued to flourish under the guidance of my father until the Second World War. Since his death I have taken up the mantle and have sought to represent the interests of Schuessler's mineral tissue salts as an adviser to the Natural Medicines Society and in writing books that make this practical and very simply system of medicine accessible to the general public. My own medical practice is based in Harley Street, where I have now enjoyed 40 years' experience of the benefits that mineral tissue salt therapy can bring to my patients.

2 Mineral tissue salts in self-medication

The history of mineral tissue salts dates from 1873, when the eminent German doctor, Wilhelm Schuessler, published the results of a series of experiments that he had been undertaking to discover the effects upon the body of the salts of some naturally occurring minerals that he had identified as important. Schuessler's work was quite revolutionary, and certainly many years ahead of its time. It is only in the last few decades that we have really begun to understand the vital importance to health of minute quantities of minerals. Much has yet to be discovered in this field.

Schuessler's method was to administer his mineral salts and then to observe any effects upon health. His theory was that many ailments were caused by imbalances of certain vital minerals in the cells of the body. Redress this imbalance, and the ailment would be cured as the cell balance was restored.

Over many years of work and study, Schuessler identified 12 vital mineral salts, and it is the administration of these, singly or in combination with one another, that is the basis of mineral tissue salt therapy that we use today.

The terms explained

In order to understand this natural system of medicine, we must first deal with a few of the terms that I shall be using throughout this book.

First, the mineral tissue salts act 'biochemically'. This word is derived from the Greek work 'bios' meaning life, therefore biochemistry is concerned with the chemistry of life, i.e. what is happening in the cells of our bodies. The cells form the 'tissue' of the body.

The word 'salt' is, of course, one with which we are all familiar. However, the use of the word here has nothing at all to do with common table salt. A 'salt' is a name for a type of compound. Thus, magnesium is a mineral used in Schuessler's mineral tissue salt therapy but it is actually taken in combination with phosphorus as a salt, magnesium phosphate. Occasionally, you may see mineral tissue salts referred to as 'cell-salts' or even as 'Schuessler salts'.

The preparation of mineral tissue salts – the homoeopathic method

The 12 tissue salts that Schuessler identified are prepared and administered in a very special way. Wilhelm Schuessler was also interested in homoeopathy, and therefore chose to administer his salts in homoeopathic doses.

The method of manufacture, along the classical principles of homoeopathic preparation laid down by the father of homoeopathy Samuel Hahnemann, is described in detail at the end of this book. The essence of the homoeopathic method of preparation is to dilute the active ingredient with lactose. The proportions used are nine parts of lactose to one part of the active mineral salt. The resultant mixture is then ground together for a considerable time and once more diluted by adding nine parts lactose to the mixture.

This whole process of successive grinding and dilution with lactose is repeated until the final product is obtained. It is a lengthy and labour-intensive process. At the New Era mineral tissue salt manufacturing plant in Humberside, which I will describe later, it takes 42 hours of continuous grinding and dilution to make every little tablet!

In homoeopathy, each successive dilution is called trituration.

With every trituration, the potency of the medicine is *increased*. The greater the dilution, the higher the potency. Most commercially available mineral tissue salts are triturated six times, with a one-in-ten dilution. It is usual to shorten this to 6x (x being the Roman numeral meaning 10).

The theory of potentization

It is worth dwelling on the theory behind homoeopathic preparations for a moment, since it is so different from the view normally taken by science.

In conventional medicinal practice, the dose is increased in proportion to the activity required. To use a simple example, you may take one paracetamol tablet if you are suffering from a mild headache, but would probably take three tablets if the headache was very severe. Exactly the same principle applies in the administration of drugs by a doctor. The doctor is trained to assess the severity of the medical problem presented to him or her, and then to administer a relevant dosage. The more severe the symptoms, then usually the higher the dose given.

Now, in homoeopathy, the exact opposite applies. A mild or moderate remedy may be given at a potency of 6x, but a homoeopathic doctor may judge that particular symptoms may require stronger medicine and will give 12x, i.e. medicine diluted a further six times. Naturally, such a contradiction is treated with contempt by many 'scientists'. 'How can it possibly be more active', they argue, 'when hardly any of the original substance remains present?'. The response is that in truth we do not know why homoeopathic products become potentized in this way, but clinical usage over almost a century has proven that the system works. Furthermore, the homoeopathic system does not only work in adults, where it is perfectly possible that a placebo effect is operating, i.e. because the person *believes* that the medicine will make them get better, they *do* get better. It also has a long history of success with young children, who are, of course, unaware that they are being given a medicine and therefore cannot possibly benefit from any placebo effect. The same applies to the use of homoeopathic preparations for the treatment of animals. The animals respond to the treatment, and the more dilute the medicine, the more potent it becomes.

Homoeopathy and mineral tissue salts

What, then, is the relationship between the systems of homoeopathy and mineral tissue salts which act biochemically? The two have a great deal in common, and many believe that biochemic mineral tissue salts are really a branch of homoeopathy. Certainly the method of preparation is similar and many of the 'Schuessler salts' are also used in standard homoeopathic remedies. However, whereas homoeopathy uses a great range of active substances, biochemistry uses only those inorganic salts that occur naturally in the body.

Dr Schuessler describes the biochemic action thus: 'My method of cure is based on the physiological chemical process, i.e. the disturbances occurring in the motion of the molecules of the inorganic substances in the human body are *directly* equalized by means of homogeneous substances, while homoeopathy attains its curative ends in an indirect way by means of *heterogeneous* substances.'

Clearly, there are differences of theory, and similarities of preparation and administration. There is a further important similarity. Both systems rely upon the close observation of the patient's symptoms to decide upon the correct therapy. Homoeopathy places a great deal of emphasis upon the building of a symptom picture of the patient. The individual remedy is given to suit individuals and their particular conditions, and is not directed solely at an illness. For this reason, the prescribing of homoeopathic medicines is a skilled business requiring close observation of the patient and then the selection of the correct preparation and potency for that patient.

Mineral tissue salt therapy is directed at an illness. Diagnose the illness by recording the symptoms and then administer the mineral tissue salt or combination of mineral tissue salts that has been found to correct the cellular imbalances causing the symptoms to occur. It is therefore very well suited to the self-treatment of common family ailments.

As we shall discover later on, mineral tissue salts are very safe to use and are therefore very suited to self-treatment by people who wish to try an alternative to standard drug therapy. Let us not dwell any further upon the similarities and differences of the two theories. I personally see no quarrel between them, and indeed use both in my medical practice. Schuessler's natural system of medicine may also help *you*. The remainder of this book is therefore dedicated to helping you to choose the correct preparation and to take it in the correct dosage. I trust that the understanding of this remarkable medical system will open up new horizons for you in the way that you care for your health.

There are a large number and variety of mineral tissue salts available today, which will be suitable for most of your needs. In the next two chapters we will go on to describe the two types of mineral salts, single tissue salts and combination tissue salts.

3 The single mineral tissue salts

The single mineral tissue salts are the 12 mineral salts that Wilhelm Schuessler originally identified as being vital in his trials. These are usually sold at 6x potency and are numbered from 1 to 12, the order being their Latin names in alphabetical order. It is this Latin name that historically has been used to indicate that the product has been homoeopathically prepared, to differentiate it from the usual chemical name of minerals when they have not been ground finely by the trituration process. For example, salt No. 12 is the mineral silicon dioxide, but when triturated it is called *Silicea* and the 6x designation indicates the level of such trituration. In most cases the Latin name is shortened to make it easier to handle.

When buying the remedies, it is only necessary to look for the number and the first name listed, to be sure that you have the right one. My own personal preference is to use the products of the New Era Company. This company has been making mineral tissue salts for over 30 years, and manufactures to a very high standard. In the New Era range, all the 12 single tissue salts are clearly numbered and are sold in light-blue tubs.

Using the single tissue salts

Now we will consider each of the 12 mineral tissue salts in turn. As you will see, together they represent a comprehensive medicine chest for the home.

No.	Name	Full Latin name	Mineral name	Formula
1	Calc. Fluor.	*Calcarea fluorica*	Calcium fluoride	CaF_2
2	Calc. Phos.	*Calcarea phosphorica*	Calcium phosphate	$Ca_3(PO_4)_2$
3	Calc. Sulph.	*Calcarea suphurica*	Calcium sulphate	$CaSO_4$
4	Ferr. Phos.	*Ferrum phosphoricum*	Iron phosphate	$Fe_3(PO_4)_2$
5	Kali. Mur.	*Kali muriaticum*	Potassium chloride	KCl
6	Kali. Phos.	*Kali phosphoricum*	Potassium phosphate	K_2HPO_4
7	Kali. Sulph.	*Kali sulphuricum*	Potassium sulphate	K_2SO_4
8	Mag. Phos.	*Magnesia phosphorica*	Magnesium phosphate	$MgHPO_4.7H_2O$
9	Nat. Mur.	*Natrum muriaticum*	Sodium chloride	$NaCl$
10	Nat. Phos.	*Natrum phosphoricum*	Sodium phosphate	$Na_2HPO_4.12H_2O$
11	Nat. Sulph.	*Natrum sulphuricum*	Sodium sulphate	$Na_2SO_4.10H_2O$
12	Silica	*Silicea*	Silicon dioxide	SiO_2

The above table lists the 12 single mineral salts in order.

No. 1 (Calc. Fluor. 6x)

In nature this occurs, as do all the other minerals, in the earth and in the rocks. In the body it occurs in:

bones
teeth
walls of blood vessels and all connective 'holding' tissues
Thus deficiency of this salt leads to upset of the above body components. Remember that these can of course lead in turn to other upsets if neglected. Thus more than one salt may be needed to be given in a particular case, but Calc. Fluor. is the one to use for maintaining tissue elasticity. The chief indications for Calc. Fluor. are as follows:

varicose veins
varicose ulcers
piles
over relaxed tissues
flabbiness
   or giving way and sagging of tissues, e.g. hernias and
   prolapse
poor teeth
late development of teeth in infants and children
deficient enamel

No. 2 (Calc. Phos. 6x)

This mineral occurs in bones and teeth and also in soft tissues but is mainly concerned with bony structures generally. Deficiency of this salt is seen in the following conditions:

slow healing of fractures
bony deformities
delay in teething and general teething problems
some types of anaemia (calcium is important for the proper
   formation of blood)
poor nutrition and digestion
coldness
cramps
chilblains
liability to colds and catarrh
children outgrowing their strength
chronic tonsillitis

some skin diseases (catarrhal type)
polypus
coccydynia
hypochondriasis (with Kali. Phos. No. 6)

In several of the above, including the latter, other remedies should often also be used. This will be covered later when I deal with the New Era combination remedies.

With a Calc. Phos. deficiency state, subjects are usually made worse by coldness, coffee, tobacco, and excessive self-contemplation of symptoms. This latter factor of hypochondriasis is due to the fact that the phosphorus balance is essential for the proper functioning of the nervous system. See No. 6 Kali. Phos. 6x later and the remedy *Nervone*.

Calc. Phos. subjects are usually helped by dry, sunny weather and by rest – preferably bed rest.

No. 3 (Calc. Sulph. 6x)

In the body this mineral occurs in connective tissue, as a blood constituent and also in the liver cells. The function in the latter case is the removal of worn out blood cells from the circulating blood. A deficiency of Calc. Sulph. impairs this cleaning activity and related problems arise as well as disorders of connective tissue. With a Calc. Sulph. deficiency the following conditions are seen:

pimples during adolescence
boils
skin eruptions
skin slow to heal
catarrh
dandruff
falling hair
vertigo with nausea
sore lips
gum boils
neuralgia
frontal headaches (particularly so in elderly people)
pancreatic upsets

liver upsets (with No. 11 Nat. Sulph. 6x)
kidney upsets

No. 4 (Ferr. Phos. 6x)

This salt is found in all the tissues of the body, but mainly in the red blood cells. The iron is concerned with the oxygen-carrying capacity of the blood. Its use in muscular coats of blood vessels becomes apparent when the effects of deficiency are seen – this leads to relaxation of the walls of blood vessels which in turn leads to congestion and inflammation. Thus Ferr. Phos. is used for all inflammations, that is all ailments ending with 'itis', e.g. bronchitis. Thus Ferr. Phos. 6x will be helpful in the first stages of these ailments and if the condition is beyond this stage then Kali. Mur. 6x should be used as well (see later).

Ferr. Phos. is a great children's remedy. It is helpful in healing their so often worrying conditions and can frequently help to put these right before the condition has advanced to the stage of diagnosis in the orthodox sense. But, as with all conditions, always see your doctor if there is the slightest doubt.

To summarize, Ferr. Phos. 6x is used in the following conditions.

    all the minor respiratory disorders
    childhood illnesses (e.g. measles, scarlet fever, etc.)
    first stage of all inflammations and fevers
    congestions
    haemorrhage
    nose bleed
    excessive periods
    throbbing, congested headache
    inflammatory rheumatism
    coughs and colds
    chills, 'feverishness'
    chestiness (in alternation with Kali. Mur. 6x)

This remedy regulates the bowel – that is from either looseness or from constipation – and is most useful in children in this respect.

Ferr. Phos. is the most frequently used of the tissue salts traditionally, but now closely followed by Kali. Phos. 6x (see later) in these stressful times.

A little powdered Ferr. Phos. 6x (they are easily crushed to a powder) when applied externally can help staunch blood flow from small cuts and promote clean and rapid healing.

No. 5 (Kali. Mur. 6x)

A deficiency of this salt affects the fibrin in the body, that is the layer below the skin that exudes thus producing the picture seen in the second stage of inflammation. Kali. Mur. is thus used for the second stage of all inflammatory illnesses. The salt is used for the following conditions:

second stage of inflammation of all 'itis' illnesses

minor respiratory disorders

coughs, cold symptoms, wheeziness

chestiness (in alternation with Ferr. Phos. 6x for children's feverish colds)

prior to vaccination or immunization to help eliminate undesirable side-effects

chickenpox

scarlet fever

mumps

measles

white/grey coating of tongue

catarrh

eczema – especially infantile

warts

acne

constipation (in liverish states and in pregnancy)

diarrhoea due to fatty foods

piles

menorrhagia (but always see your doctor)

leucorrhoea

shingles

burns

scalds

With a Kali. Mur. 6x deficiency state, patients usually find they are worse with fatty foods.

No. 6 (Kali. Phos. 6x)

Kali. Phos. 6x is the remedy for the nervous system and is the great nerve soother – phosphorus being the chief nerve mineral. It is used for all nervous disorders and those that are so often called 'neurotic' illnesses, and treating them along these lines is most helpful. From the presence of Kali. Phos. in other tissues of the body come its uses in the following conditions:

all temporary nerviness
melancholia
hysteria
highly strung
fearfulness
despair
timidity and shyness
loss of mental and nerve power
nervous debility
emotional strain
excessive blushing
neuritis
incontinence or retention of urine from *nervous* causes
nightmares – all 'unjustified' fears, e.g. of water
inability to sleep
nervous indigestion
nervous diarrhoea
nervous headache
alopecia
nervous asthma
menstrual colic – spasms, cramps etc.
ineffectual labour pains from anxiety
sexual incompetence and frigidity

Patients requiring this remedy are usually made worse by noises and moving about, and when left alone too long, and also by over-excitement. They are helped by soothing company and conversation on uncontroversial topics.

The remedy is useful at some stage in most illnesses, e.g. for the lack of sleep and panic so often seen; indeed it can be very useful for the relatives of patients who may very well need the help of a salt almost as much as the patient.

No. 7 (Kali. Sulph. 6x)

This tissue salt is found in the external layers of epithelial membrane, such as the skin, and maintains skin condition. Disturbance of this causes yellowish catarrh and shedding of surface epithelia. It is thus concerned with the third stage of inflammation of all inflammatory illnesses – the 'itis' diseases. It is also concerned with oxygen carriage in the body. Kali. Sulph. is used for the following conditions:

third stage of all inflammations
bronchitis
yellow coating of tongue
thick yellow mucous catarrh
whooping cough
gastric catarrh
intestinal catarrh
asthma
colic (if response to Mag. Phos. is poor)
menstrual disorders
to help maintain healthy hair
dandruff
foul breath
measles
eczema
psoriasis
brittle nails
minor skin eruptions with scaling or sticky exudation
flashes of heat and chilliness
giddiness of inflammatory type
palpitations
headache

Patients requiring Kali. Sulph. are frequently worse in hot weather.

No. 8 (Mag. Phos. 6x)

Mag. Phos. is found in similar tissues to Calc. Phos. 6x, i.e. bones, teeth and nerve tissues, as well as in blood vessels and muscles, but basically it is a soft tissue salt. Deficiency of this salt leads to cramp-like conditions and collicky states and so it is known as the anti-spasmodic tissue salt.

Mag. Phos. is used for the following conditions:

muscle cramps and spasms
minor occasional pains
hiccups
spasmodic shivers and twitching
intermittent retention of urine and bladder spasm
enlarged prostate
writer's cramp and similar conditions
stuttering
crampy labour pains
painful menstruation
ovarian neuralgia
gallstone colic
kidney stone colic
teething in infants
constipation in infants
flatulence
intercostal neuralgia
headaches
toothache when pains are sharp, shooting, boring
rheumatic pains
neuralgia generally

Mag. Phos. subjects are often lean, nervous people. Pains are usually worse from cold and touch and helped by warmth, pressure and bending.

No. 9 (Nat. Mur. 6x)

Nat. Mur. is based on a mineral called sodium chloride, or common table salt. We need one gram of the crude salt per day in Britain but the average intake is 10 grams daily. This excessive intake creates havoc with many people, and the fine particle minerals of tissue salt remedy No. 9, that is Nat. Mur. 6x, helps to put right the sodium imbalance in the body.

Nat. Mur. occurs in all tissue fluids in the body and is often regarded as the most important of the 12 salts. It is a distributor and controller of water throughout the body. Nat. Mur. is used in the following conditions:

circulation problems
shock
watery vomiting
diarrhoea
minor haemorrhage
anaemia (always see your doctor)
watery colds with flow of tears and runny nose
loss of smell
loss of taste
prolapse (with Calc. Fluor.), e.g. shingles, herpes and blisters
insect stings and bites generally
thin watery milk in lactation
excessive size of breasts in pregnancy
hydrocele (in the scrotum)
excessive tears
excessive salivation
teething with excessive salivation
water brash
sneezing
hay fever
influenza
asthma
constipation (dry stools)
headaches (early morning type)
hysteria
sterility
nettle rash
chronic eczema
acne
greasy skin
ulcer of gums
gout
sciatica
sunstroke

No. 10 (Nat. Phos. 6x)

This salt occurs in the intercellular fluids and in the body tissues generally. It has two main types of action in the body. It controls acid generally, sometimes called the 'acid neutralizer', and it helps deal with fatty acids.

Its first action has its uses in dealing with uric acid and lactic acid etc., thus helping to prevent or treat acid states.

The second main function is seen in the help it can give in dyspepsia due to excessive intake or improper usage of fat.

Nat. Phos. 6x is used for the following conditions:

    all acid states of the bloodstream 'uric acid dialysis'
    rheumatism of joints
    rheumatic arthritis
    gout
    acid taste
    to help prevention of gallstones etc.
    sick headaches
    giddiness
    conjunctivitis
    itching of nose
    red, blotchy face
    sea sickness (with Kali. Phos.)
    sour breath
    grinding of teeth during sleep
    yellow coated tongue
    catarrh and thick yellow mucus
    heartburn
    nausea
    morning sickness of pregnancy
    gastric indigestion
    sour flatulence
    loss of appetite
    constipation
    diarrhoea
    acidity
    incontinence from acidity
    sterility from acidity
    leucorrhoea – sour smelling

sleeplessness from itching in acid states

rheumatic pain tendency

Subjects requiring Nat. Phos. are made worse by fats and sugars (sweets in children). Reducing their intake is usually found helpful.

No. 11 (Nat. Sulph. 6x)

This salt occurs mainly in the intercellular tissues, and it has an effect on the water content of the body, but in a rather different way from Nat. Mur. – Nat. Sulph. appears to withdraw water and so it helps the elimination of effete cells. Nat. Sulph. is used mainly in the following conditions:

to help with the body water balance

biliousness of watery nature

vomiting in pregnancy

diarrhoea

constipation

tongue grey or greenish/brown

bitter taste

liver upsets

gall bladder upsets

kidney upsets

pancreatic upsets

rheumatism in watery subjects

gout in watery subjects

asthma of a watery nature

bronchial catarrh

flu symptoms

hay fever

warts

ear noises and earache from fluid retention

flatulence and colic

distended stomach

queasiness

digestive upsets

hydrocele (in the scrotum)

Subjects needing Nat. Sulph. are usually worse in damp weather, and feel better in dry conditions, hot or cold.

No. 12 (Silica 6x)

This salt occurs in the connective tissue, and disturbance of its balance affects the nervous system from its presence in the coverings of nerve fibres. Disturbance of the silica content of the body usually ends in pus formation and Silica 6x helps to promote and push out such pus (note that Calc. Sulph. has a rather different action). Therefore Silica 6x can be thought of as a conditioner and a cleanser. It is also a preventative in premature ageing – a lack of this salt causing premature ageing by atrophy of tissues.

In our food, silica is found in wholemeal bread and is the 'grit' of our diet.

Silica 6x is used in the following conditions:

> lack of 'grit' (i.e. stamina both physical and mental)
> absent-mindedness
> poor memory (see Kali. Phos.)
> foot sweats
> sweats generally if of an unpleasant nature
> alcoholic intolerance
> falling out of hair
> brittle nails (in alternation with Kali. Sulph.)
> eye strain
> asthma from dust
> pimples and spots
> styes
> fissures
> boils
> chronic bronchitis
> coccydynia
> alopecia
> whitlows
> ingrowing toe-nails
> premature ageing

Patients needing silica are usually worse at night and suffer from feet becoming cold. They are usually helped by a warm atmosphere and hot baths.

This concludes the list of the twelve tissue salts. To take them follow the instructions on the container or follow the advice of a homoeopathic physician. You cannot take an overdose – more than the body needs would just be a waste and nothing more, so there is total safety.

This, then, is the full list of the 12 single tissue salts. Each product has an abbreviated list of the main indications written on it to guide you to the right one. Dosage instructions will also be found on the tub, although I will be dealing with the dosage in detail in a later chapter.

4 The combination mineral tissue salts

In reading the list of uses for single mineral tissue salts, you may have noticed that in a number of cases the same ailment was mentioned under two or three headings. Many years of clinical experience and observation have resulted in the formulation of a range of combination remedies, i.e. remedies that contain three or four single mineral tissue salts. These are formulated to deal with a specific ailment, and should prove to be very effective. They are, of course, easier to use than taking a number of single tissue salts.

Combination remedies are manufactured in the same way as single remedies, the homoeopathic methods described earlier being strictly adhered to. The correct mixture of mineral salts is first prepared and then this mixture is triturated to the 6x potency.

The New Era Company makes a comprehensive range of combination remedies by these methods. These combinations have become so popular that they are now the standard formulations, and it is these which I shall describe. The remedies are readily available from all health food shops and from most of the larger chemists.

The combination remedies: A to S

There are 18 combination remedies. For simplicity, each one is given a letter, which is clearly marked on the container, along with the indications for use of the product. Thus, for example, combination J is marked 'chestiness, colds, coughs'. They are sold in colour-coded tubs.

The following list shows the mineral tissue salts contained in each combination remedy and the main uses for the product. A more extensive coverage of use is included in the therapeutic index later in this book.

Combination Remedy A

This remedy contains the tissue salts Ferr. Phos. 6x, Kali. Phos. 6x, and Mag. Phos. 6x. It is used for: sciatica, neuralgia and neuritis.

Combination Remedy B

This remedy contains the tissue salts Calc. Phos. 6x, Kali. Phos. 6x and Ferr. Phos. 6x. It is used for: general debility, edginess, nervous exhaustion and convalescence.

Combination Remedy C

This remedy contains the tissue salts Mag. Phos. 6x, Nat. Phos. 6x, Nat. Sulph. 6x and Silica 6x. It is used for: acidity, heartburn, and dyspepsia.

Combination Remedy D

This contains: Kali. Mur. 6x, Kali. Sulph. 6x, Calc. Sulph. 6x, Silica 6x. It is used for: minor skin ailments, scalp eruptions, eczema, acne and scaling of the skin.

Combination Remedy E

This contains: Calc. Phos. 6x, Mag. Phos. 6x, Nat. Phos. 6x, Nat. Sulph. 6x. It is used for: flatulence, colicky pains and indigestion.

Combination Remedy F

This contains: Kali. Phos. 6x, Nat. Mur. 6x, Silica 6x. It is used for: nervous headaches and migraine.

Combination Remedy G

This contains: Calc. Fluor. 6x, Calc. Phos. 6x, Kali. Phos. 6x, Nat. Mur. 6x. It is used for: backache, lumbago, piles.

Combination Remedy H

This contains: Mag. Phos. 6x, Nat. Mur. 6x, Silica 6x. It is used for: hay fever and allied conditions.

Combination Remedy I

This contains: Ferr. Phos. 6x, Kali. Sulph. 6x, Mag. Phos. 6x. It is used for: fibrositis and muscular pain.

Combination Remedy J

This contains: Ferr. Phos. 6x, Kali. Mur. 6x, Nat. Mur. 6x. It is used for: coughs, colds, and chestiness and is the autumn and winter seasonal remedy.

Combination Remedy K

This contains: Kali. Sulph. 6x, Nat. Mur. 6x, Silica 6x. It is used for: brittle nails and falling hair.

Combination Remedy L

This contains: Calc. Fluor. 6x, Ferr. Phos. 6x, Nat. Mur. 6x. It is used for: sedentary lifestyle, toning the tissues and is a natural tonic.

Combination Remedy M

This contains: Calc. Phos. 6x, Kali. Mur. 6x, Nat. Phos. 6x, Nat. Sulph. 6x. It is used for: rheumatic pains.

Combination Remedy N

This contains: Calc. Phos. 6x, Kali. Mur. 6x, Kali. Phos. 6x, Mag. Phos. 6x. It is used for: menstrual pain.

Combination Remedy P

This contains: Calc. Fluor. 6x, Calc. Phos. 6x, Kali. Phos. 6x, Mag. Phos. 6x. It is used for: aching feet and legs.

Combination Remedy Q

This contains: Ferr. Phos. 6x, Kali. Mur. 6x, Kali. Sulph. 6x, Nat. Mur. 6x. It is used for: catarrh and sinus disorders.

Combination Remedy R

This contains: Calc. Fluor. 6x, Calc. Phos. 6x, Ferr. Phos. 6x, Mag. Phos. 6x, Silica 6x. It is used for: infant's teething pains.

Combination Remedy S

This contains: Kali. Mur. 6x, Nat. Phos. 6x, Nat. Sulph. 6x. It is used for: stomach upsets, biliousness, queasiness, sick headaches. This is an excellent summer seasonal remedy.

Further special combinations

There are some further special combinations of the mineral tissue salts that have been formulated for particularly troublesome conditions. Again, these are very readily available and may be extremely helpful if you suffer from the particular problem at which they are aimed.

Elasto

This contains Calc. Fluor. 6x, Calc. Phos. 6x, Ferr. Phos. 6x and Mag. Phos. 6x. *Elasto* has a very big and loyal following of people who use it for troublesome conditions of the legs. In particular, *Elasto* may be used for tired and aching legs and varicose veins. It derives its name from its benefits to the elastic tissues in the body.

Nervone

This contains Calc. Phos. 6x, Kali. Mur. 6x, Kali. Phos. 6x, Mag. Phos. 6x and Nat. Phos. 6x. The formulation may be used for nerve pains and for nervous disability. *Nervone* is a safe and reliable remedy for a whole range of 'nerve troubles' and allied ailments.

Zief

This contains Ferr. Phos. 6x, Nat. Phos. 6x, Nat. Sulph. 6x and Silica 6x. *Zief* is an effective remedy for the treatment of rheumatic conditions.

Conclusion

As you will have now learned, there is a considerable and comprehensive range of single and combination mineral tissue salts available for use in most common ailments. The remainder of this book is devoted to showing you how to select the correct remedy for a given condition, and how to use it to the best advantage.

5 How to use mineral tissue salts

The great advantage of using the mineral tissue salt therapy is that it is, at the same time, both safe and flexible. No other system offers users such a degree of control over the dosage and administration of the therapy. It is a very different system from conventional medicine, but once the principles are mastered, the benefits will become obvious.

Dosage

The first principle to be grasped is that there is no single correct dose for mineral tissue salts. The amount that you take is more dependent upon the type of symptoms and the severity of them.

In adults, an average dosage regime would involve taking four tablets three times a day in divided doses. (Dosages for children need to be reduced. Advice is given in a later chapter in this book.) If symptoms are very severe, the frequency of the dosage may be increased to perhaps four tablets every hour, and then gradually tailed off as the symptoms subside.

As an example of a typical therapy, let us imagine that you are suffering from a severe attack of catarrh. Your nose is blocked and you feel an uncomfortable pressure within your head. Combination Q is an excellent remedy for relieving this condition. You may therefore take four tablets at 9.00 a.m., when the symptoms are very bad. The four tablet dosage is again repeated at 10.00 a.m.

and 11.00 a.m. By midday you are gaining relief and may not feel the need to take another dose until perhaps 1.00 p.m., with another at 6.00 p.m. and a final dose for the day at 10.00 p.m. The next day you are feeling a little better, but still need to keep the symptoms under control. You therefore drop back to three doses of four tablets, one in the morning, one at midday and one in the evening.

This regime may be necessary for perhaps two or three days, after which you feel that you can further reduce the dose to maybe three tablets three times a day or only take one four tablet dose twice a day. When all symptoms have disappeared, it is essential to continue to tail off the therapy for two or three days to ensure that there is no 'rebound' effect as soon as the therapy is stopped.

Some indications, such as rheumatism or nervous conditions, may need a slightly different approach. Here you may find it beneficial to undertake therapy at low doses for a number of weeks, increasing the dose or frequency if the symptoms become troublesome. In these cases, for example, a dose of perhaps two tablets twice a day may be adequate to control the symptoms, but four tablets could be taken, or the frequency of doses increased to three to five times a day, if the condition becomes especially troublesome. Again, dosages and frequency of taking the tablets should be tailed off when symptoms diminish.

Remember, you cannot take an overdose of mineral tissue salts. They are quite safe. What you need to do is to develop a sensible regime of treatment that suits you. Everyone is different. We have different metabolisms and our ailments are not the same as everyone else's. Therefore, you will need to experiment to find the best level of dosage and frequency to suit you. This is the great benefit of mineral tissue salt therapy. You are in complete control of the therapy; and since you are using small amounts of active materials taken frequently, you are in control of the medicines entering your body.

So, to recap, the principles of dosage are as follows:

- Four tablets – three doses during the day is the standard adult dose.
- Take tablets hourly if the symptoms are severe.

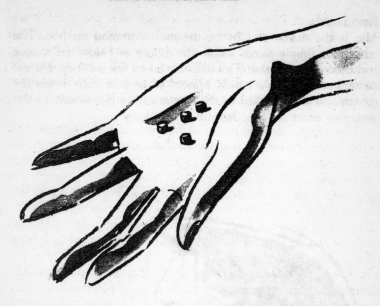

- Tail off the dosage and frequency as symptoms improve.
- Continue the therapy for at least three days after symptoms have ceased.
- For longer-term problems, use lower doses of tablets and increase dosage or frequency if symptoms are troublesome. Tail off therapy in the usual way or resume the original 'maintenance' dose.

How to take mineral tissue salts

Mineral tissue salts may be taken with or without food. There is also no problem with taking tea or coffee before or after the therapy. This differs from the normal practice with homoeopathic medicine, where patients are often advised not to take remedies half an hour before or after food.

There are a number of ways of taking the mineral tissue salt tablets:

By mouth

This is the easiest and by far the most common method. The tablets are simply placed inside the mouth or below the tongue and allowed to dissolve. This will only take a few seconds. *There is no need to swallow the tablets.* Mineral tissue salts 'melt' inside the mouth and are absorbed by the mucus within the mouth. In this way, they enter the bloodstream very quickly.

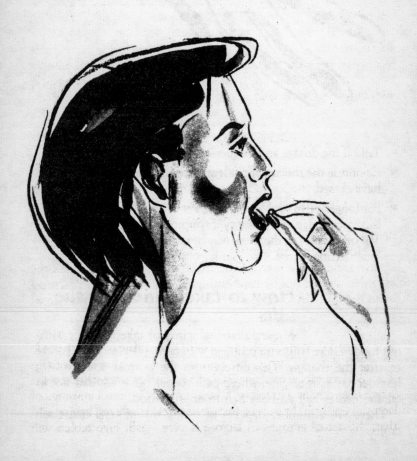

As we will mention later, this 'melting' property makes mineral tissue salt therapy extremely suitable for children, who are often very unwilling to swallow tablets. Mineral tissue salt tablets are tasteless and can simply be popped under the tongue of a child. Ten seconds later they will have melted and the medicine is within the child's system and doing its work. What could be more simple!

Ointment or paste
Occasionally, the tablets may need to be made into a paste for external application. This can easily be achieved by crushing 10–20 tablets into a powder and then mixing in a small amount of boiled water.

In solution
Mineral tissue salts may be crushed and given in a solution of boiled water or milk. Instructions for this method, for example adding it to a bottle feed, are given in chapter 11.

Some questions and answers

1. Can I use mineral tissue salts during pregnancy?
Yes. As always, you should be very careful in taking any medicines during pregnancy. However, mineral tissue salts are safe, and I have never encountered any problems in this area.

2. How long can I keep the tablets?
Usually the manufacturers recommend that, after opening, the pot of tablets should not be kept for more than three years. You must store them in dry conditions and (very importantly) away from sunlight.

3. I am lactose-intolerant. Will the tablets upset me?
The first thing to say is that mineral tissue salt tablets contain lactose. Each tablet contains 0.07g of lactose as the carrier for the active ingredients. Therefore, if you are upset by small amounts of lactose you should not take these remedies. However, having said that, the actual amount of lactose is very small. Five tablets will

contain 0.35g of lactose. Put another way, this is the same amount as in a thimbleful of milk. Quite often, this small amount of lactose will give no trouble. If in doubt, my advice is not to take the remedies.

4. I am taking other drugs from the doctor. Will mineral tissue salts affect them?

No. There is usually no problem. Mineral tissue salts work in a different way from conventional medicines and there is no clash. If in doubt, consult your local doctor or pharmacist.

5. Can I take more than one type of mineral tissue salt at a time?

Yes. It is safe and is very often recommended. For example, if you had a high temperature accompanied by a runny nose, I would recommend taking Ferr. Phos. (No. 4) together with Nat. Mur. (No. 9) at the dosage of three tablets each three times a day until the symptoms have subsided.

Combination mineral tissue salts of course combine three to five of the single salts together in one tablet.

6. I have tried a particular mineral tissue salt, but the symptoms did not improve. What am I doing wrong?

There are many possible causes. First, I would recommend checking the treatment. In the therapeutic index later in this book I have listed more than one treatment for some conditions. If the first is not helpful, you may benefit from the second choice listed. The most frequent problem is failure to continue with the therapy for long enough. Remember, mineral tissue salts work in a slow and gentle way. It is a drop-by-drop approach. It is no use expecting miracles after just one dose. Persevere with your own 'course' of treatment in the way I described at the beginning of this chapter. Many ailments, for instance rheumatism, may require several months of regular, steady treatment to get them under control. Mineral tissue salts are not 'blockbuster' drugs. They work within the body to restore the cell balance gradually. It is these imbalances which cause the symptoms of the illness. We are administering minute quantities of the minerals vital to cell balance. It may take time to restore the balance, especially if the problem has persisted for some time. My advice is to be patient and persistent.

7. Are there any side-effects?

No. The active ingredients are administered in minute quantities and are very unlikely to cause any side-effects. If you think that you have side-effects, see your doctor. It may be something that needs further medical attention.

8. I am diabetic. Should I take mineral tissue salts?

The tiny amount of milk sugar present in mineral tissue salts (0.07g per tablet) should be of no concern to diabetics. If, however, you are concerned, do consult your doctor.

Some case histories

The following are a few examples of the benefits of using mineral tissue salt therapy.

Stress

Mr T. S., aged 53, was made redundant two years ago, and after six months found further employment. But then that firm collapsed, so he is now out of work with no job prospects at all. This caused him so much stress that he was put on tranquillizers by his doctor, the latter being a family friend and full of understanding.

However, the patient was fearful of tranquillizers, and so he had prescribed for him *Nervone*, which made all the difference. He is now, with some confidence, taking steps to be self-employed. He feels his position has changed from one of hopelessness to one in which he is taking action himself in a positive way, and he puts the reason for the change down to his use of *Nervone*.

In so many cases, the stresses and strains of life can respond to mineral tissue salts.

Pregnancy prescribing

Mrs A. S., aged 34, wanted to become pregnant but had not conceived after ten years of marriage. Investigation of the couple had indicated that all was physically well with them both. But it did seem that she was obviously in great distress from her inability to have a child.

She took mineral tissue salt No. 6 (Kali. Phos.) to help her relax, and mineral tissue salt No. 2 (Calc. Phos.) to help improve the general health of her body. She became pregnant after four months of treatment, and continued with the tissue salt Calc. Phos. throughout the term of the pregnancy. This helped to provide her with extra cover for her health and that of the baby. The birth was excellent, the baby was breast-fed, and now she is a

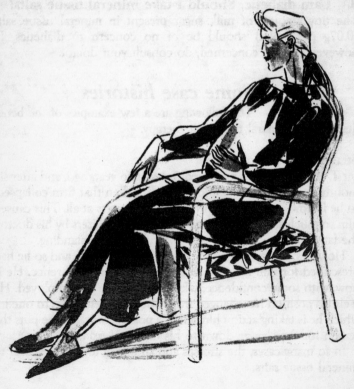

toddler and the mother happily pregnant again. During teething, the baby was helped with mineral tissue salt combination R.

This illustrates the fact that it is perfectly safe to take these mineral tissue salts throughout pregnancy, and also that they are suitable for babies, toddlers and indeed all age groups, not just adults.

Abdominal symptoms

Irritable bowel syndrome is fairly common and has no really satisfactory treatment along orthodox lines. The four mineral tissue salts Calc. Phos., Mag. Phos., Nat. Phos. and Nat. Sulph. can be very helpful indeed in this condition. This particular group of remedies is found in Combination E.

6 Care of the whole person

In order to cope with today's 'pace of life', each one of us has to take responsibility for the well-being of our whole body, not just treating parts in isolation when they go wrong.

Stress and strain caused by a build-up of pressure at work or at home, or both, can often cause illnesses when our bodies' defences are at a low ebb. Therefore, a different attitude should be adopted to provide a way of life to combat the effects of wear and tear on our minds and bodies.

Attention should be paid to the daily diet, whenever possible eating whole food, reducing meat and increasing fish. Plenty of green and root vegetables should be eaten daily, including regular salads (i.e. raw vegetables). Also, plenty of fresh fruit as an alternative to sweets and cakes, and you should reduce your intake of salt as there is usually enough in food and from the cooking process.

It is important not to be overweight, as carrying around these extra pounds puts extra strain on the heart. Eat everything that's healthy and appetizing, but in small quantities. Chew food thoroughly and eat it at a leisurely pace, making meal time a relaxing social occasion – this not only makes one feel fuller, but also helps the nutrients from the food to be absorbed more thoroughly. When recovering from an ailment, then a light, easily digestible, diet is required; fish, milk, eggs and root vegetables provide the best nutrients and are easily eaten and digested.

Sufficient exercise is extremely important – a brisk walk a day provides fresh air and, by exercising the lungs, improves breathing,

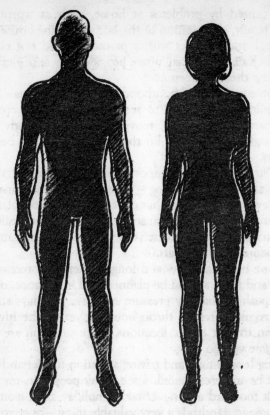

not to mention toning up the muscles of the body. When I say a 'brisk' walk, I do mean walking at a reasonably fast pace – what the Americans refer to as 'race walking'.

Everyone should regularly appraise their way of life, including work and most importantly leisure time. Particular attention should be paid to planning leisure time – this should be as well planned as your work time.

If your job involves working under constant pressure, resulting in stress from time to time, then take Kali. Phos. (No. 6) to combat the pressure. Having an organized approach to your workload can be very helpful in relieving the psychological problem of being over-worked and harassed.

Stress caused by problems at home, such as worries about children/family, organization of the home, moving house (buying and selling) and troubles with a partner, should not be under-estimated. Kali. Phos. can often provide safe and gentle relief when facing these problems.

The home and its neighbourhood can cause problems – this situation should be scrutinized to see if a solution that creates less pressure can be reached, e.g. moving from a particularly noisy or violent neighbourhood can lift the pressure that one bears from day to day.

When stressed, it is very important not to increase alcohol consumption and turn to smoking – the short-term effect may feel as if it is relieving the problem, but dependence on alcohol, smoking and caffeine for a prop can cause harmful long-term health problems. Also alcohol can increase your weight, which in turn creates more pressure on your heart.

Everyone needs holidays and long weekends to recharge their batteries, and these should be planned well in advance, otherwise they get pushed aside by pressure of work. Holidays should be taken at regular intervals throughout the year to healthy places. If you plan to visit exotic locations, make sure you are in good health *before* you go.

Planning leisure time and paying attention to diet and exercise must not be underestimated. I see many people in my practice who work too hard and never take a holiday, then wonder why they become ill. Health is a very valuable thing – once ruined, no amount of money can buy it back again. Therefore, it is advisable to take care of not just parts of the body but the whole person.

7 Hints on the relief of hay fever

There is no cure for hay fever, but if you, or anyone in your family, suffer from this seasonal allergy, this chapter may help. It explains exactly what hay fever is, and gives some useful hints on a lifestyle that could help you to cope more easily, plus some sensible ideas about diet.

The advice in this chapter is relevant to all hay fever sufferers, so please take time to read it. To help ease the discomfort of hay fever, New Era's hay fever remedy is the natural choice for very young children to take. It does not cause drowsiness and it will not conflict with any other medication. In order to reduce hay fever symptoms in the peak of the season New Era's hay fever remedy combination H should be taken as early as possible, i.e. starting from the beginning of April, to increase resistance later.

Hay fever is such a common complaint that most people know its symptoms. You have to have experienced an attack, though, to realize just how wretched the sneezing, runny nose and itchy eyes can make you feel. To make matters worse, treatment can occasionally compound the problem. Decongestant nasal sprays and drops tend to lose their effect after several days of continuous use, and can also harm the delicate lining of the nasal passages, making the symptoms worse.

Certain, although not all, antihistamine drugs have strong sedative effects. This is the last thing you want if you are studying for exams and needing to feel not only physically fit but mentally alert and able to concentrate.

As all hay fever sufferers know, attacks are commonest and most severe during the months of late spring and early summer. This is also the time when students are most likely to be sitting important examinations. If performance is not to be marred by watery eyes, sneezing and sniffing attacks, or a blocked, stuffy nose, you must get to know what triggers your attacks and what preventative measures you can take.

Hay fever is a form of rhinitis, meaning inflammation of the lining of the nose. It is seasonal and due to an allergy to pollen. Approximately four million people in the U.K. are thought to suffer from it, and there is a tendency for hay fever to run in families. Men are affected more than women, although the reason for this is unknown.

Pollen allergy can appear at any age, but tends to be worst among teenagers and young adults. Some people get symptoms for five or six consecutive seasons and then never have another attack, while others suffer season after season for up to 20 years or more. A small minority of sufferers go on to develop bronchial asthma and/or nasal polyps (swellings in the mucous lining of the nose).

Symptoms

Attacks generally start suddenly. Frequently sneezing is associated with an intense itch inside the nose, occasionally more on one side than on the other. The feeling has been compared to having sniffed itching powder or hot chilli pepper, as the mucous membranes feel 'hot' as well as irritating. Some people develop lines across the lower parts of their nose from habitually rubbing its tip to relieve the itching.

Soon after the irritation starts, watery fluid begins to flow freely down the nose, making frequent wiping a necessity. Even with the use of soft tissues, the repeated skin friction can make the sensitive area around the nostrils and upper lip sore, red and chapped.

Itchy, watering eyes and a tickling feeling in the throat are also frequent symptoms. Bright lights make matters worse, and the tendency to rub the eyes makes them swollen and bloodshot.

Soon, a blocked nose and the necessity to breathe through the mouth, at least partly, complete the picture.

Hay fever symptoms can last from a few hours to several days, depending upon the weather, the pollen count and other factors such as the sufferer's emotional state, stress level and general state of health. If you are familiar with these problems, you will know how easily they can lead to irritability, fatigue and depression, and what a handicap they can become when you are studying.

Causes

Strictly speaking, only allergy to pollen can produce hay fever. This is why 'hay fever proper' occurs only during the pollen-producing months of spring and summer. Some people suffer from hay fever symptoms all the year round, and this condition, known as perennial rhinitis, is considered in a later section.

Every year, several thousands of tons of tree and grass pollen are released into the air during the spring and summer months. It is in this way that pollen, produced by plants for the purpose of fertilization, is able to reach its required destination of another plant of the same species.

The wind is responsible for much pollen transport, however, and it is windborne pollen that causes hay fever. Highly coloured and strongly scented flowers rarely play a significant part in this process. This is because they attract insects, and are pollinated by the insect population that visits them. It is the lighter and more buoyant pollen of trees, grasses and weeds that is more likely to cause symptoms.

Plantain and other common weeds are often responsible for hay fever symptoms. Once one of these pollens causes you allergy problems, the rest are likely to do so as well. That is why hay fever often starts as early as March, and continues until July or August.

Spring hay fever is caused mainly by tree pollens, and the more severe summer variety by grass pollens, with weed pollens triggering symptoms in the late summer and autumn. Pollen (and mould spores) follow a seasonal pattern year after year, but vary with geographical location.

The quality of pollen produced depends upon the weather,

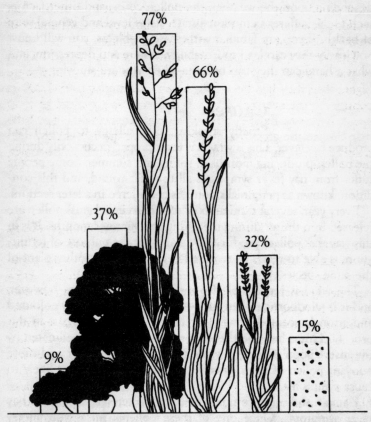

77%

66%

37%

32%

15%

9%

APRIL MAY JUNE JULY AUGUST SEPTEMBER

TREE POLLENS   MOULD SPORES
ARE COMMON   ARE COMMON

GRASS POLLENS
ARE COMMON

symptoms tending to be worse on hot, dry, windy days. This is the reason why hay fever tends to affect sufferers most severely during June and July. These are the months when the grass pollens are most prolific. Hay fever is responsible for about four million lost working days per year in the U.K. This about twice the number of working days lost as a result of industrial injuries.

The weather, in fact, plays an important part in the production of pollen grains. In 1986, for example, the pollen counts were higher than they had been for 21 years, registering over 1,000 in contrast to the average of 190. A pollen count of more than 50 causes hay fever. Experts believe that the very cold spring of 1986 first delayed the growth of flowers, and that the subsequent mild weather made many species of flowers bloom simultaneously, thereby releasing masses of pollen grains.

Perennial rhinitis

This is a closely associated condition, producing much the same symptoms as hay fever. In all, it is estimated that about six million people in the U.K. (that is, a tenth of the population) are affected. Sufferers complain of having an almost permanent head cold, but it is necessary only to experience symptoms for an hour or more out of 24, on most days of the year, for perennial rhinitis to be diagnosed. So distressing can the perpetual sneezing, nose blowing, eye irritation and nasal stuffiness become that it is understandable that sufferers feel as though they are never free from them.

The most prominent symptom in perennial rhinitis is nasal blockage, affecting five out of ten sufferers. Sneezing and watery nasal discharge affect three out of ten sufferers, but eye symptoms and an itchy throat are less common in many cases of this condition than they are in pollen-allergy hay fever.

Hay fever can cause perennial rhinitis during the spring and summer months. Allergic rhinitis due to causes (allergens) other than pollen also accounts for many cases. These include fungal spores, animal dander (scurf) and house dust.

While it is an excellent idea to consult your doctor about troublesome hay fever and perennial rhinitis symptoms, there are a number of things that you can do to alleviate your symptoms in a natural, drug-free way, which will in no way conflict with any treatment your doctor may prescribe. It is even possible to reduce the frequency with which you experience your attacks, if you are willing to take a little time and trouble sorting out your own 'trigger factors'. Whatever your job or lifestyle, this is well worth aiming at. If you are a student faced with weeks of revision and important exams, it could make all the difference to your results and to your future.

Lifestyle hints

For allergic rhinitis, including hay fever, prevention is in most cases better than cure. Here are some ways of avoiding some of the more common allergens.

- Keep a daily record of your symptoms and compare this with the pollen count. You will soon get to know whether your 'hay fever' is really due to pollen allergy.

- If you are affected in this way, avoid open fields and freshly mown lawns, however inviting.

- Try to stay indoors when the pollen count is high.

- Wearing dark glasses if you must go out on dry, warm, breezy days will help to protect your eyes.

- If animals affect you, avoid visiting friends with cats or dogs and, if you have pets yourself, keep them out of your bedroom at all times.

- House dust may be your problem – dust and vacuum daily, not forgetting soft furnishings and curtains, which should be washed or dry-cleaned monthly.

- The minute organism called the house dust mite, living within house dust, is responsible for much allergic rhinitis. They are too small to be seen, and tend to inhabit mattresses, pillows and other bedding. A sheet of plastic film over your mattress may help. Always air beds daily too, by stripping them right back and exposing the bottom sheet to the fresh air. Keep bedroom windows at least partly open always, unless pollen is your problem.

- Deep freeze your pillows! The house dust mite dies at temperatures lower than 10°C. Simply rotate the pillows you use, through your freezer, allowing several hours for them to 'thaw out' before you re-use them.

- Never use feather mattresses, pillows or duvets.

- Turn the central heating off in your bedroom, at least during the night. Try increasing the humidity in the various rooms you use during the day, by placing a bowl of water in each room.

- Experiment with ventilation, too, to find out what suits you best.

Diet

A change of diet is found by many sufferers to help. A balanced, wholefood diet that avoids junk foods and additives will improve your overall state of health and resistance to stress, whatever the allergen causing your attacks. When the chemical additives in processed foods or other dietary items are themselves to blame, improvement is often dramatic.

I would recommend hay fever sufferers to drink mineral water and diluted, freshly squeezed fruit and vegetable juice for the first two days of an attack, and for a light diet to be followed for several days thereafter. By this, I mean fresh fruit and raw vegetables, with herb tea or spring water to drink.

The avoidance of mucus-forming foods is also thought of highly as a form of hay fever treatment. These foods include white flour and white sugar and their products; refined, processed foods, including 'doctored' cereals; fried food, animal fats and dairy products; chocolate; cocoa; salt and tea; coffee and alcohol.

Emphasis should be placed upon raw or lightly cooked fresh fruit and vegetables; wholewheat flour and its products; nuts; eggs; fish; and white meat.

8 *Minerals and trace elements*

Most people are aware of the need for vitamins in their diet, but there is another group of vital substances that are essential for normal life. These substances are the minerals and elements. Although nearly everyone recognizes the importance of calcium and iron, some 20 minerals are known to have important roles in the human body. These nutrients cannot be synthesized by the body and must be supplied by the foods we consume, whether of animal or vegetable origin. These foods are derived from the soil or the sea, the chemical compositions of which depend on the rocks that lie beneath them.

Minerals are usually divided into the *major elements*, such as calcium, magnesium and sodium, and the *trace elements*, examples of which are iron, zinc, copper, iodine and fluorine. These trace elements are needed in very much smaller quantities than the major elements. Nevertheless, both groups are equally important for maintaining good health. Minerals have the following three main functions:

- They are components of many enzymes and other proteins such as haemoglobin.
- They occur as soluble salts controlling the composition of the body's fluids and cells.
- They are important constituents of our bones and teeth.

Optimum health cannot be achieved unless all the essential minerals, as well as all the other required nutrients, are available. Good nutrition means an adequate intake of all these nutrients, and it is therefore essential that a wide range of different foodstuffs is consumed by eating a little of everything, but not too much of anything.

Suggested levels of intake for only two mineral elements, calcium and iron, have been established in the U.K. These are known as the recommended daily amount or RDA. The RDA is an estimate of the amount of any nutrient each person should consume daily, and provides assurance that the needs of almost all healthy individuals will be met. There are, however, certain conditions, such as pregnancy, lactation, or some disease states, in which there will be a greater requirement by the body for nutrients. Although the other minerals have not yet been given an RDA, they are still important. Minerals such as calcium, magnesium, phosphorus, iron and sodium are the best understood. The amounts needed of the others are so small that it is only recently that they have been capable of being measured.

Minerals are somewhat unique amongst the dietary nutrients in that they are relatively poorly absorbed from the foods we consume. Whereas the other nutrients are absorbed efficiently, most minerals achieve only between 5% and 15% absorption. The exceptions are sodium, potassium and chlorine, which average almost 100% absorption. One factor that can affect the availability of minerals is dietary fibre. The presence of fibre in the diet is important because a certain amount promotes normal function of the intestinal tract and because it may assist in the elimination of toxic substances from the body. However, a substance called phytic acid is associated with fibre, and this can bind minerals in the gut, making them unavailable for absorption. In addition, minerals can be removed from foods during processing and refining processes although unlike vitamins they are not destroyed. These factors, together with an increased demand at certain times may lead to shortages that could be restored by the sensible use of supplements.

The roles of some minerals are briefly on the following three pages.

Calcium

Calcium is the most abundant mineral in the body and, together with phosphorus and magnesium, it is important as a structural component of bones and teeth. It also plays a vital role in blood-clotting and the transmission of nerve impulses to control muscle movement. The main food sources are dairy products, white bread and all bakery products made with white flour. This is because white flour is fortified with the mineral. In order to absorb and utilize calcium (and phosphorus) properly, an adequate level of vitamin D is essential. A deficiency of calcium or of vitamin D can cause rickets in children. Poor calcium intake throughout life, especially if this occurs in women, may give rise to the brittle bone condition, osteoporosis. This is a result of a loss of calcium, and therefore of bone. The rate of loss is accelerated in women during and immediately following the menopause, and is partly responsible for the prevalence of bone fractures in many old people. It is therefore important to ensure that adequate levels of calcium are consumed throughout life. High-fibre diets can inhibit the absorption of calcium, as can diets high in phosphates or containing high levels of protein. It may therefore be recommended to take a calcium supplement, especially when few dairy products and only wholemeal bread are consumed.

Iron

Over half the body's iron is in the form of haemoglobin, the oxygen/carbon dioxide-carrying protein of the blood. A dietary deficiency results in anaemia, a condition characterized by tiredness, lethargy and breathlessness. In addition, any loss of blood from the body increases the demand for iron. In view of this, the requirement for women in their reproductive years is larger than for men. The best dietary sources are liver, meat and eggs, the iron present in these foods being referred to as organic iron. The mineral, in the inorganic form, is also found in vegetables, bread and cereals, and its absorption is enhanced by vitamin C. Some reports have suggested that an increased susceptibility to infections may occur when iron deficiency exists.

Zinc

Virtually all body tissues contain some zinc, but especially the liver, kidneys, brain and pancreas. It is an important component of many enzymes and is necessary for proper growth and development. Food content of zinc varies greatly, although it is widely distributed. Zinc from foods of animal origin is more efficiently absorbed by the body. A deficiency may lead to delayed wound healing, reduced appetite and lack of physical, mental and sexual development. Low levels of dietary zinc are reported to be associated with both acute and chronic infections, and supplementary zinc is suggested to help the symptoms of the common cold. Food processing reduces the content and availability of the mineral.

Magnesium

Most of the magnesium is present in the bones, but it is also an important component of some enzymes and is essential for neuromuscular function. It is important for growth, maintenance and repair of the body, and works as a co-factor for the functioning of vitamin B6. Magnesium is widespread in foods, especially those of vegetable origin.

Selenium

Selenium is an antioxidant and often works together with vitamin E. Food content of selenium varies widely, depending on the levels present in the soil. Food processing and refining markedly decrease these levels. Selenium may be important in maintaining the immune system, may protect against toxic metals and may have an anti-inflammatory effect. Epidemiological evidence suggests that selenium may have a protective action against cancer, and it could be of value to arthritis sufferers.

Chromium

Chromium is involved in the utilization of glucose and is therefore essential for the maintenance of blood sugar levels. The richest sources are brewer's yeast, molasses, cheese, liver and wheatgerm, but the absorption of chromium by the body is poor. Epidemiological studies have suggested that chromium deficiency may be a factor in certain types of heart disease.

Copper

Copper is widespread amongst foods, liver and shellfish being the richest sources. It is an essential component of various enzymes, is important for healthy blood formation and may be involved in the development of resistance to illnesses. A deficiency may contribute towards anaemia, but an excess can be harmful.

Combating deficiency

We tend to become deficient in these essential minerals because our food is now grown on soils that, by successive cropping, have been depleted of these minerals. It is not normal farming practice to put them back in the form of fertilizers, which are now mainly chemical. A small range of minerals is made by New Era Laboratories Ltd.

1. Lead-free dolomite

This is a very logical, natural and safe source of both calcium and magnesium – and you need no hesitation in taking it in the recommended dosage if you think you may have a deficiency of either calcium or magnesium.

2. Zinc with copper

This is a natural and safe way to supplement your diet with these two essential substances in an easy-to-take form.

3. Multi-trace minerals

As I have shown, we need a large number of trace elements in our diet but, unfortunately, many people may tend to be deficient in one or other of the elements zinc, manganese, chromium, calcium and selenium. These tablets are available with or without iron.

9 *Therapeutic Index*

These next pages are designed to give a quick reference to the correct mineral tissue salt to be used for given indications. Where more than one remedy is shown, then the remedies are given in order of preference. For example, under the heading 'Arthritis' you will find *Zief*, Combination M and Combination I listed. All of these remedies have been found to be helpful in alleviating the symptoms of arthritis. However, I would recommend *Zief* as a first choice, reserving Combinations M and I in case *Zief* should not prove to be effective.

General conditions

If symptoms persist or you are worried about the condition, consult a qualified person.

Conditions	Remedies
Abdomen, bloated	Combination E, No. 8 (Mag. Phos.)
Aches and pains (general)	Combination G, Combination A, Combination M (especially rheumatic pains)

Conditions	Remedies
Aching feet or legs	*Elasto*, Combination P, No. 1 (Calc. Fluor.)
Acid regurgitation	Combination S, No. 10 (Nat. Phos.)
Acidity (heartburn)	Combination C, No. 8 (Mag. Phos.)
Acne	Combination D, No. 3 (Calc. Sulph.)
Anaemia	No. 4 (Ferr. Phos.), Combination B
Anxiety	*Nervone*, No. 6 (Kali. Phos.)
Arthritis	*Zief*, Combination M, Combination I
Asthma	Combination J, No. 6 (Kali. Phos.)
Backache	*Zief*, Combination G, No. 1 (Calc. Fluor.)
Bad breath	Combination C, No. 10 (Nat. Phos.)
Bed wetting	No. 6 (Kali. Phos.)
Biliousness	Combination S, No. 5 (Kali. Mur.)
Blisters	No. 9 (Nat. Mur.)
Bloodshot eyes	Combination H, No. 4 (Ferr. Phos.)
Boils	Combination D, No. 3 (Calc. Sulph.)
Bronchitis	Combination J, No. 4 (Ferr. Phos.)
Burns (to aid recovery)	No. 5 (Kali. Mur.), Combination D, Combination M
Catarrh	Combination Q, No. 7 (Kali. Sulph.)
Chapped hands	No. 3 (Calc. Sulph.), Combination P
Chapped lips	Combination P, No. 1 (Calc. Fluor.), No. 3 (Calc. Sulph.)
Chestiness	Combination J, No. 5 (Kali. Mur.)
Chilblains	No. 2 (Calc. Phos.), Combination P
Chills	Combination B, No. 4 (Ferr. Phos.)

Conditions	Remedies
Circulation (poor)	No. 2 (Calc. Phos.)
Colds	Combination J, No. 4 (Ferr. Phos.)
Colic	Combination E, No. 8 (Mag. Phos.)
Constipation	Combination S, No. 9 (Nat. Mur.)
Coughs	Combination J, No. 4 (Ferr. Phos.)
Coughs (acute or irritable)	Combination J
Coughs (convulsive bouts)	Combination H
Cramp	Elasto, No. 8 (Mag. Phos.)
Craving for food	Nervone, No. 6 (Kali, Phos.)
Cystitis	No. 6 (Kali. Phos.)
Dandruff	Combination D, No. 7 (Kali. Sulph.)
Depression and despondency	Nervone, No. 6 (Kali. Phos.)
Diarrhoea	Combination S, No. 5 (Kali. Mur.)
Digestive upsets	Combination C, No. 11 (Nat. Sulph.)
Drowsiness	Combination F, No. 12 (Silica)
Dry skin	Elasto, No. 1 (Calc. Fluor.)
Dysmenorrhoea	Combination N, No. 8 (Mag. Phos.)
Dyspepsia	Combination C, No. 10 (Nat. Phos.)
Earache	No. 1 (Calc. Fluor.), No. 7 (Kali. Sulph.)
Eczema	Combination D
Eyes water	Combination Q, Combination H, No. 9 (Nat. Mur.)

Conditions	Remedies
Fever	Combination I, No. 4 (Ferr. Phos.), No. 8 (Mag. Phos.)
Fibrositis	Combination I, No. 4 (Ferr. Phos.)
Flatulence	Combination E
Flu	Combination J, No. 10 (Nat. Sulph.)
Gout	Zief, Combination A
Gum boil	Combination C, No. 12 (Silica)
Haemorrhoids	Elasto, No. 1 (Calc. Fluor.)
Hay fever	Combination H, No. 8 (Mag. Phos.)
Headache (nervous)	Nervone, Combination F, No. 6 (Kali. Phos.)
Headache (sick with gastric upset)	Combination S, No. 11 (Nat. Sulph.)
Headache (with pains)	Combination F, Combination I, No. 8 (Mag. Phos.)
Heartburn	Combination C, No. 11 (Nat. Sulph.)
Hiccups	Combination E
Hoarseness	Elasto, No. 2 (Calc. Phos.)
Hysteria	Nervone, No. 6 (Kali. Phos.)
Incontinence	Combination B, No. 6 (Kali. Phos.)
Indigestion	Combination E, No. 8 (Mag. Phos.)
Inflammation	Combination L, Combination I
Influenza	Combination J, No. 4 (Ferr. Phos.)
Irritability	Nervone, No. 6 (Kali. Phos.)
Itching	Combination P, No. 6 (Kali. Phos.), No. 2 (Calc. Phos.)
Laryngitis	Combination J, No. 2 (Calc. Phos.)
Lethargy	Combination L
Lumbago	Combination G, Combination A

Conditions	Remedies
Menstrual pain	Combination N, No. 8 (Mag. Phos.)
Migraine	Combination F, No. 11 (Nat. Sulph.)
Minor skin complaints	Combination D, No. 7 (Kali. Sulph.)
Moody, anxious	Nervone, No. 6 (Kali. Phos.)
Morning sickness	Combination S, No. 10 (Nat. Phos.)
Muscular pain	Combination I, Combination M, No. 8 (Mag. Phos.)
Nails (brittle)	Combination K, No. 7 (Kali. Sulph.)
Nails (inflammation around)	Combination L, No. 4 (Ferr. Phos.)
Nasal catarrh	Combination Q, Combination H, No. 4 (Ferr. Phos.)
Nasal discharge	Combination J, No. 9 (Nat. Mur.)
Nausea	Combination S, No. 10 (Nat. Phos.)
Neck (stiffness)	Zief, Combination M, No. 4 (Ferr. Phos.)
Nerves	Nervone, No. 6 (Kali. Phos.)
Nettle rash	Combination L, No. 1 (Calc. Fluor.)
Neuralgia	Nervone, No. 2 (Calc. Phos.)
Neuralgia (aggravated by cold)	Combination A, No. 8 (Mag. Phos.)
Neuralgia (with periods)	Combination N, No. 8 (Mag. Phos.)
Nightmares	Nervone, No. 6 (Kali. Phos.)
Nose bleed	No. 4 (Ferr. Phos.)

Conditions	Remedies
Palpitations (nervous)	Nervone, Combination B, No. 6 (Kali. Phos.)
Periods (heavy)	Elasto, No. 4 (Ferr. Phos.)
Periods (painful)	Combination N, No. 8 (Mag. Phos.)
Periods (scanty)	Combination L, No. 9 (Nat. Mur.)
Pharyngitis	Combination R, No. 2 (Calc. Phos.)
Phlegm (thick)	Zief, No. 12 (Silica)
Phlegm (watery)	Combination J, No. 9 (Nat. Mur.)
Piles	Elasto, No. 1 (Calc. Fluor.)
Pimples	Combination D, No. 3 (Calc. Sulph.)
Psoriasis	Combination D
Queasiness	Combination S, No. 10 (Nat. Phos.)
Rheumatic pains	Zief, Combination M, No. 4 (Ferr. Phos.)
Rhinitis	Combination J, No. 9 (Nat. Mur.)
Run down	Combination L
Sciatica	Zief, Combination A, Combination M
Sedentary lifestyle	Combination L, No. 1 (Calc. Fluor.)
Shivering	Elasto, No. 2 (Calc. Phos.)
Sickness (vomiting)	Combination C, No. 10 (Nat. Phos.)
Skin (dry)	Combination K, No. 7 (Kali. Sulph.)
Skin (greasy)	Combination C, No. 10 (Nat. Phos.)
Skin (scaling)	Combination D, No. 7 (Kali. Sulph.)
Skin (spots)	Combination D

Conditions	Remedies
Skin (wrinkled)	Elasto, No. 6 (Kali. Phos.)
Sleepiness	Combination L, No. 9 (Nat. Mur.)
Sneezing	Combination Q
Sprains and strains	Combination I, Combination P, No. 4 (Ferr. Phos.)
Stings (insects)	No. 9 (Nat. Mur.)
Stomach upsets	Combination S, No. 11 (Nat. Sulph.), No. 10 (Nat. Phos.)
Taste (loss of)	Combination Q
Taste (unpleasant)	Combination C, No. 11 (Nat. Sulph.)
Teething	Combination R, No. 2 (Calc. Phos.)
Throat (from speaking or singing)	Elasto
Throat (sore)	Combination J, No. 4 (Ferr. Phos.)
Throat (sore and dry)	Combination J, No. 9 (Nat. Mur.)
Throat (tickling in)	Elasto, No. 1 (Calc. Fluor.)
Throat (ulcers in)	Combination C, No. 3 (Calc. Sulph.)
Tongue (blisters on)	Combination Q, No. 9 (Nat. Mur.)
Tongue (coated)	Combination C, No. 10 (Nat. Phos.)
Tongue (inflamed)	Combination Q, No. 4 (Ferr. Phos.)
Tonsils (inflamed)	Combination Q, No. 4 (Ferr. Phos.)

Conditions	Remedies
Toothache	No. 8 (Mag. Phos.)
Travel sickness	Combination F, Combination S, No. 10 (Nat. Phos.), No. 6 (Kali. Phos.)
Ulcers (corner of mouth)	Combination D, No. 12 (Silica)
Ulcers (mouth)	Combination C, No. 10 (Nat. Phos.)
Vaginal Discharge (coloured)	Combination B, No. 6 (Kali. Phos.)
Vaginal Discharge (white)	Combination D, No. 5 (Kali. Mur.)
Varicose veins	Elasto, No. 1 (Calc. Fluor.)
Vertigo	Nervone, Combination S, No. 6 (Kali. Phos.)
Warts	Combination D, Combination K
Weakness (convalescence)	Combination B, No. 2 (Calc. Phos.)
Wheeziness	Combination Q, No. 5 (Kali. Mur.), No. 4 (Ferr. Phos.)

10 *Female conditions*

Below is a list of conditions in women, and their remedies. Note that New Era remedies can be used during pregnancy.

Conditions	Remedies
Aching feet and legs	*Elasto*, No. 1 (Calc. Fluor.)
Backache during pregnancy	Combination G; Combination A at end of final weeks
Cystitis	No. 6 (Kali. Phos.), No. 5 (Kali. Mur.); Nervone – nervous; Combination N if infection
Dysmenorrhoea	Combination N, No. 8 (Mag. Phos.)
Frigidity	*Nervone*, No. 6 (Kali. Phos.), No. 8 (Mag. Phos.)
Menopausal symptoms	
Hot flushes	No. 4 (Ferr. Phos.), No. 6 (Kali. Phos.)
Irritability	*Nervone*, No. 6 (Kali. Phos.)
Run down	Combination L

Conditions	Remedies
Menstrual pain	Combination N, No. 8 (Mag. Phos.); No. 6 (Kali. Phos.) covering pre-tension and aching at period
Morning sickness	Combination S or No. 10 (Nat. Phos.)
Periods	
Heavy	*Elasto* or No. 4 (Ferr. Phos.)
Painful	Combination N, No. 8 (Mag. Phos.)
Scanty	Combination L, No. 9 (Nat. Mur.)
Pimples	Combination D
Pregnancy	*Elasto*, No. 2 (Calc. Phos.); to minimize stretch marks, take from 6 months till 1 month after delivery
Sedentary lifestyle, varicose veins	Combination L and *Elasto* around the ankles
Vaginal discharge	
White	Combination D
Coloured	Combination B CHECK WITH DOCTOR

11 *Therapeutic index for children*

        Families today have to be able to move around the country, either where work can be found or where their employers ask them to go. It is not unusual for a mother with a young family to find herself in a strange town or city without her mother or friend or relative to turn to for advice and comfort about some of the problems that, she feels, may seem trivial to a total stranger.

This can lead to a feeling of isolation and, coupled with uncertainty about which medications can now safely be given to children to soothe and ease symptoms, even a minor illness such as a cough or cold can add to the already stressful demands of coping with a family.

Self-help is now actively encouraged by doctors on straightforward problems and what could be a safer method of self-help than homoeopathically prepared mineral tissue salts. After a century's experience any harmful side-effects would have been reported, but none have been recorded from New Era's active ingredients. If the body cells are not deficient of minerals, then the excess of mineral tissue salts will simply be excreted – therefore you cannot overdose on these remedies.

If your children have an intolerance to milk, then it does not automatically imply that they are intolerant to lactose, which is the milk *sugar* contained in homoeopathic remedies. The protein in milk is very often the cause of this intolerance. Protein is not present in lactose and is, therefore, not present in New Era homoeopathic preparations. The milk sugar should be of no concern to diabetics, as the small amount normally consumed should cause no harm. If you need more information, refer to your doctor.

As New Era homoeopathic preparations are non-addictive, free from harmful side-effects, cannot be overdosed and dissolve easily on the tongue with no unpleasant after-taste, they are ideal for treating the everyday ailments of children.

New Era remedies are suitable for all ages of children including babies from about three months old, as they find them very easy to take with no large tablets to swallow.

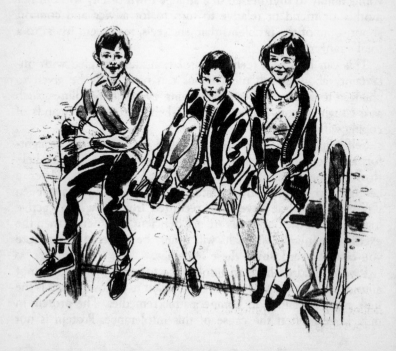

Dosage for babies and children

Press the tablet(s) into a powder and put into the baby/toddler's mouth with a spoon or as a solution in a spoon – this can be rubbed around the gums. For babies the dose should be one tablet (with each feed) six times a day. For toddlers the dose is two or three tablets three times a day. When they are of nursery school age, give four tablets three times a day. From the age of six years onwards, the dose is five tablets three times a day.

Children's ailments

I now list the common ailments of children, and their remedies.

Conditions	Remedies
Bed wetting	No. 6 (Kali. Phos.), No. 4 (Ferr. Phos.), Combination B
Colic	Combination E or No. 8 (Mag. Phos.)
Constipation	Combination S or No. 5 (Kali. Mur.)
Baby	Two or three tablets at each feed
Toddler	Adult dose
Cries easily	No. 6 (Kali. Phos.)
Diarrhoea	Combination S or No. 5 (Kali. Mur.) – normal adult dose
Earache	No. 1 (Calc. Fluor.), No. 7 (Kali. Sulph.) – Combination J and Combination N call a doctor
Hyperactivity	No. 6 (Kali. Phos.)
Inflamed tonsils	Combination Q
Itching and scratching	Combination P

Conditions	Remedies
Poor appetite	Combination B – check with a doctor
Skin rashes	Combination D
Teething	Combination R or No. 2 (Calc. Phos.) as often as possible (every half hour); rub into gums with finger
Travel sickness	Combination F and Combination S – before and during journey
Vomiting	Combination E; No. 2 (Calc. Phos.) – if continues, call a doctor

12 Therapeutic index for pets

Almost everyone at some time in their life has kept or wanted to keep a pet – particularly a dog or a cat. The main reason for this is the company, interest and affection that they can provide. The family pet is totally dependent on us, and we must do our best to understand and fulfil its needs, providing to the best of our ability a happy and healthy life for our pet.

Domesticated animals cannot choose their own food, and depend on their owners to provide them with a well-balanced diet. The nutrients required are proteins, carbohydrates, fats, minerals, vitamins and water. Dogs and cats seldom suffer from a deficiency in the quantity of food but deficiency in the quality is much more common.

Caring for our pets properly means that we have to provide good-quality food plus a supplement for a glossy coat, plenty of fresh air and exercise together with regular grooming. People who like to use a natural, homoeopathically prepared remedy for themselves also like to treat their pets with this safe system of medicine.

Administration of the dose of mineral tissue salts is as follows:

Dogs – to lick tablets off the hand; cats – crush tablet and sprinkle on food.

The following list of ailments can be treated with New Era mineral tissue salts.

Conditions	Remedies
Anal gland (inflamed)	No. 4 (Ferr. Phos.) and No. 12 (Silica) – vet to clear gland
Appetite (repressed)	No. 6 (Kali. Phos.)
Bad breath	Combination C and No. 10 (Nat. Phos.)
Bladder inflammation (cystitis)	No. 4 (Ferr. Phos.) and No. 9 (Nat. Mur.)
Bronchitis	Combination J
Canker	No. 10 (Nat. Phos.) in addition to veterinary treatment
Catarrh	Combination Q
Constipation	Combination S and No. 9 (Nat. Mur.)
False pregnancy	No. 6 (Kali. Phos.)
Fits	No. 6 (Kali. Phos.)
Flatulence	Combination E and No. 10 (Nat. Phos.)
Fur ball	Combination S and No: 11 (Nat. Sulph.)
Gastritis	Combination C
Hair loss	No. 10 (Nat. Phos.)
Interdigital cysts	Combination D
Nervous conditions	No. 6 (Kali. Phos.), Nervone
Poor coat (dandruff)	Combination B
Rheumatism	Combination M and Combination I
Skin complaints	Combination D
Travel sickness	Combination F and Combination S

Appendix:
The New Era
factory in Hull

Whilst writing this book, I visited the modern homoeopathic manufacturing unit recently built by New Era Laboratories, now based in Hull, North Humberside.

I was most impressed by the standard of hygiene in the new building, which is referred to by company staff as 'tablet and grinding'. It was also refreshing to find such a watertight and rigorously enforced procedure of quality control.

As the New Era manufacturing unit is the only one in the U.K. producing moulded homoeopathic tablets, I thought it would be interesting to describe the manufacturing and quality-control processes of New Era mineral tissue salts summarized from my tour.

Starting from the beginning, all materials and packaging materials, as they arrive on site at the factory, are put into quarantine. Each ingredient is then sampled by the quality control inspector and sent to the laboratory for analysis. Once this has been carried out it is checked against the ingredient specification set by New Era and the certificate of analysis from the suppliers or manufacturers. The product is released only if it meets all the criteria and then, and only then, it is moved into the main stores to be used for production. Each product has a method of manufacture, formulation and finished product specification, all of which constitute the product documentation and controls.

The lactose powder has to be of British Pharmacopoeia standard, which ensures its purity. It is weighed according to the manufacturing formula, witnessed by the quality control inspector, and then the control sheets are signed indicating that all ingredients and quantities are correct. The active ingredients, which are the pure minerals, are weighed in the quality-control laboratory on electronic balances to ensure the accuracy of the weight, then issued to production to add to the lactose.

The grinding mills are kept running throughout the process of trituration for nine hours. The intermediate is then sampled and sent to quality control for analysis. It is checked on the atomic absorption spectrometer, the sensitivity of which can go down to 0.05 parts per million. Once the intermediate is passed, it moves to the stage of preparing the 1x, 2x, all the way up to 6x dilution, which takes a total of 42 hours. After the preparation of the 6x powder, an acacia mucilage is added to the fine powder as a binder for tabletting. The acacia mucilage is first sterilized because acacia is a natural product from trees and is therefore bound to be contaminated with all sorts of organisms. Hence the sterilization process will provide us with the acacia that is organism-free, i.e., sterile.

The acacia is added and mixed in clean stainless-steel mixers and the whole powder, which is now ready for tabletting, is moved to the tabletting area. The latter is under a controlled atmosphere supplied by filtered air. The moulded tablets are then passed through hot electric ovens to dry them and make them hard.

Samples are taken by the quality-control inspector at regular intervals during the production period to check the weight of the tablet, dimensions, thickness/diameter, rate of disintegration and active ingredients in each tablet. If these specifications fall within the limits of the finished product specification, the batch is released by quality control. Then, and only then, it moves to production for filling and packaging.

The combination remedies are prepared in the same way, using the same technique and methods, except that, after milling, depending on the ingredients in each combination, these powders are put in a blender to produce a homogeneous product. For example, if we take Combination H, a batch of Mag. Phos. is prepared, a batch of Nat. Mur. is prepared and a batch of Silica is prepared using the same technique as for the single tissue salts.

These three mineral tissue salts are then put into a blender and mixed to produce a homogeneous mix, and this will then give us combination H for hay fever. The tabletting process is exactly as for the single tissue salts.

Index

abdomen, bloated 59, symptoms 43
aches and pains, feet 60, 67, general 59
acid neutralizer 26
acid regurgitation 60
acidity (heartburn) 60, 62
acne 60
alcohol 46
anaemia 60
anal gland inflammation 74
anxiety 60, moodiness 63; see also stress
appetite, poor in children 72, repressed in pets 74
arthritis 59, 60
asthma 60

backache 60, during pregnancy 67
bad breath 60, in pets 74
bed wetting 60, 71
biliousness 60
blisters 60
blood system, constituents 19, poor circulation 61, red cells 20, varicose veins 66, 68, walls of blood vessels 18
bloodshot eyes 60
boils 60
bones 18, 24, 54, 56

British Biochemic Association 10
bronchitis 60, in pets 74
burns 60

caffeine 46
Calc. Fluor. (Calcarea fluorica) 17, 18
Calc. Phos. (Calcarea phosphorica) 17, 18–19
Calc. Sulph. (Calcarea sulphurica) 17, 19–20
calcium 55, 56, 58
canker 74
catarrh, 60, in pets 74, nasal 63
cell-salts see mineral tissue salts
chapped hands 60
chapped lips 60
chestiness 60
chilblains 60
children, ailments 71–2, dosages 71, milk intolerance 69–70, therapeutic index for 69–72; see also individual conditions
chills 60
chloride of potash see Kali. Mur.
chlorine 55

chromium 57–8
circulation see blood system
colds 61
colic 22, 61, 71
combination mineral tissue salts 30–4, A to S 30–3, Elasto 34, Nervone 19, 34, 41, Zief 34
connective tissue 19, 28
constipation 61, 71, in pets 74
convalescence 66
conventional medicines 40
copper 58, zinc with 58
coughs 61
cramp 61
craving for food 61
crying 71
cystitis 61, 67, in pets 74

dandruff, 61, in pets 74
depression and despondency 61
diabetics 41, milk sugar and 70
diarrhoea 61, 71
diet 44, hay fever and 53
digestive upsets 61
dolomite, lead-free 58
dosage 35–7
drowsiness 61

dry skin 61
dysmenorrhoea 61, 67
dyspepsia 61

earache 61, 71
eczema 61
Elasto 34
exercise 44-5
eyes, bloodshot 60,
    watering 61

false pregnancy 74
feet, aching 60, 67
female conditions 67-8; *see
    also individual conditions*
Ferr. Phos. (Ferrum
    phosphoricum) 17, 20-1
fever 62
fibre, mineral absorption
    and 55
fibrin 21
fibrositis 62
fits, in pets 74
flatulence 62, in pets 74
flu *see* influenza
fluoride of lime *see* Calc.
    Fluor.
food craving 61
frigidity 67
fur ball 74

gastritis, in pets 74
Gilbert, Dr Henry 10
gout 62
gum boils 62

haemorrhoids 62, 64
Hahnemann, Samuel 9, 12
hair loss, in pets 74
hay fever 47-53, 62, causes
    49-51, diet 53, lifestyle
    changes 52-3, perennial
    rhinitis 51-2, pollens,
    48, 50, symptoms 48-9,
    trigger factors 52
headaches 62
heartburn 60, 62
Hensel, Dr Julius 10
Hering, Dr Constantine 10
hiccups 62
hoarseness 62

homoeopathy, mineral
    tissue salts and 14-15,
    salt preparation 12-13
hot flushes 67
hyperactivity 71
hysteria 62

incontinence 62
indigestion 62
inflammation 21, 62, anal
    gland in pets 74, around
    nails 63, of tongue 65,
    of tonsils 65, 71
influenza 62
inter-cellular fluids 26
inter-cellular tissues 27
interdigital cysts 74
iron 55, 56, 58
iron phosphate *see* Ferr.
    Phos.
irritability 62, 67
itching 62, and scratching
    in children 71

Kali. Mur. (*Kali
    muriaticum*) 17, 21
Kali. Phos. (*Kali
    phosphoricum*) 17, 22-3,
    45, 46
Kali. Sulph. (*Kali
    phosphoricum*) 17, 23

lactose intolerance 39-40,
    69-70
laryngitis 62
lead-free dolomite 58
lethargy 62
liver 19
lumbago 62
Luyties, Dr H.C.G. 10

Mag. Phos. (*Magnesia
    phosphorica*) 17, 23-4
magnesium 55, 57, 58
magnesium phosphate *see*
    Mag. Phos.
manganese 58
melting property 38-9
menopausal symptoms 67

menstrual pain 22, 63, 64,
    67
migraine 63
mineral tissue salts,
    combination 30-4,
    dosage 35-7, history of
    9-10, homoeopathy and
    14-15, means of taking
    37-9, preparation 12-13,
    terms explained 11-12;
    see also individual salts
minerals 54-9, combating
    deficiency 58, fibre and
    55, multitrace 58, poorly
    absorbed 55; *see also
    individual minerals*
moodiness 63
morning sickness 63, 67
muscular pain 63

nails, brittle 63,
    inflammation around 63
nasal catarrh 63
nasal discharge 63
Nat. Mur. (*Natrum
    muriaticum*) 17, 24-5
Nat. Phos. (*Natrum
    phosphorica*) 17, 26-7
Nat. Sulph. (*Natrum
    sulphuricum*) 17, 27
Natural Medicines Society
    10
nausea 63
neck, stiffness 63
nerves 63, in pets 74;
    nervous system 22-3, 28
Nervone 19, 34, 41
nettle rash 63
neuralgia 63, aggravated by
    cold 63
New Era Company 10, 12,
    16, Hull Factory 75-7
nightmares 64
nose bleeds 64

palpitations 64
paste 39
perennial rhinitis 51-2
periods, heavy 64, 67,
    menstrual pain 63, 64,
    67, scanty 64, 67

persistence with treatment
  40
pets, therapeutic index for
  73–4
pharyngitis 64
phlegm 64
phosphate of lime see Calc.
  Phos.
phosphate of potash see
  Kali. Phos.
phosphorus 55
phytic acid 55
piles see haemorrhoids
pimples 64, 67
potassium 55
potentization 13–14
pregnancy 39, 41–3, 68,
  backache during 67, false
  in pets, 74, morning
  sickness 63, 67
preparation 12–13
psoriasis 64
pus formation 28

queasiness 64

rheumatic pains 64
rheumatism, in pets 74
rhinitis 48, 64, perennial
  51–2; see also hay fever
run down 64, 67

Schuessler, Dr W.H. 9–10,
  11, 14, 16
Schuessler salts see mineral
  tissue salts
sciatica 64
sedentary lifestyle 64, 68
selenium 57, 58
shivering 64

Shortened Therapeutics
  (Schuessler) 9
sickness 64
side-effects 41
silica (silicon dioxide) 17,
  28
skin 23, dry 61, 64,
  greasy 64, minor
  complaints 63, pets 74,
  pimples 64, 67, psoriasis
  64, rashes 72, scaling 64,
  spots, 64, wrinkled 65
sleepiness 65
smoking 46
sneezing 65
sodium 55
sodium chloride see Nat.
  Mur.
sodium phosphate see Nat.
  Phos.
sodium sulphate see Nat.
  Sulph.
soft tissue 24
sprains 65
stings 65
stomach upsets 65
storage 39
strains 65
stress 41, at home 46, at
  work 45; see also anxiety
sulphate of lime see Calc.
  Sulph.
sulphate of potash see Kali.
  Sulph.

taking mineral tissue salts
  37–9, by mouth 38 9,
  in solution 39, melting
  property 38–9, ointment

39, paste 39
taste, loss of unpleasant 65
teeth 18, 24, 54, 56,
  teething 65, 72,
  toothache 66
terms explained 11–12
therapeutic index 59–68,
  children 69–72, female
  conditions 67–8, for pets
  73–4; see also individual
  conditions
throat 65
tongue 65
tonsils 65, 71
trace elements 54–9; see
  also individual minerals
travel sickness 66, 72, in
  pets 74
trituration 13

ulcers 65–6

vaginal discharge 66, 68
varicose veins 66, 68
vertigo 66
vomiting 64, 72

Walker, Dr M. Docetti 10
warts 66
water system 25, 27
weakness 66
wheeziness 66
whole-body well-being 44–
  6, diet 44, exercise 44–5,
  stress 45–6

Zief 34
zinc 57, with copper 58